WHAT'S IN A NAME?

People's preoccupation with medical names for diseases never ceases to amaze me. These names, for particular maladies, provide convenient shorthand for the medical establishment, maybe even solace for the poor souls who find themselves in a health predicament.

Perhaps it's because people think that if someone could just give them a name for what ails 'em, there is a magic pill that will cure it.

Another Perspective

Consider this:
disease literally means: ***(dis)*** absence of, ***(ease)*** freedom from worry, pain or agitation.

An alternative for medical shorthand could be helpful. There are three states of health where people can find themselves:

HEALTHY, when the body's systems are working at peak efficiency. You know who these people are – these are people who radiate.

NOT SICK, when the body is not working efficiently and compensating for minor system shortcomings and failure. If you ask one of these people "How are you doing?" the best they can muster is "I'm OK."

SICK, when the body has lost the ability to compensate for failing systems and needs serious help.

Unfortunately, NOT SICK is the state of health for most people. It's the difference between playing catch with your son or taking a nap; going dancing or falling asleep in your chair before the news comes on the TV. You feel good enough to go to work but not bad enough to go to the doctor. Or if you do seek help you may be told not to concern yourself because "*You are just getting older.*" Or worse, "*You will just have to learn to live with it.*"

Clear Definitions and Actions

Human health complaints can be categorized as follows: *injury, infection and degeneration (imbalanced, wearing or worn-out systems.)*

The first category, <u>injuries</u>, are bumps, bruises, scrapes, cuts and broken bones. They are typically repaired with stitches and casts. Injuries can be minimized with normal caution. In fact, I believe improvements for treatment in this category contribute the most to the increased life expectancy in the United States. Thanks to improved machine safety and the changes in the way we live, fatal accidents are less prevalent.

The second category, <u>infections</u>, is caused by bugs – viruses, bacterium and fungi.

Generally, they can be minimized with good personal sanitation: keeping your hands away from your face, mouth and nose; washing your hands before eating; keeping food preparation areas clean. (Sounds like your mother talking to you doesn't it?) If you keep your body strong, your immune system can do its job. Sanitation improvements have contributed to life expectancy. Also, topical and ingested antibiotics have made a positive contribution as well;

A VIEW OF
Health

The Body's Regeneration Factory

Frank A. Lucas, PhD, cNHC

Published in the United States of America

ISBN 979-8-89395-953-6 (SC)

Frank A. Lucas Publishing
222 West 6th Street
Suite 400, San Pedro, CA, 90731
frank@nupro.net

Order Information and Rights Permission:

Quantity sales. Special discounts might be available on quantity purchases by corporations, associations, and others. For details, contact the publisher at the address above.

For Book Rights Adaptation and other Rights Permission. Call us at toll-free 1-888-945-8513 or send us an email at admin@stellarliterary.com.

This information is not intended to diagnose, treat, cure or prevent any disease. These discussions are provided for general educational purposes only and in no way should be taken as medical advice. Readers are encouraged to make health care decisions based upon personal research and in partnership with qualified health care professionals.

Table of Contents

however, their overuse may in fact have a negative impact in the long run.

Thankfully, the medical community has come to realize the benefits of antibiotics are limited to bacterial infections and are slowing their pell-mell distribution. You would be well-served knowing the source of your infection before taking an antibiotic prescription.

If you have the misfortune to experience an injury or infection, it isn't the end of the world. A little professional intervention, some time to heal and you're generally as good as new.

The third category of dis-ease is degeneration of the body. It is not as clear cut as the first two categories.

Degeneration is a murky combination of medical definitions (diagnoses) and actions (prescriptions) – when in fact it is a direct reflection of how well people care for their bodies.

I'm not talking about slathering oil on your skin; I'm talking about the quality and quantity of the fuel you put in the regeneration and regrowth factory you call your body. The equation is very simple – garbage in, garbage out. In a nutshell, this can be the land mine that gets all of us!

The Body is a Regeneration Factory.

The factory analogy is right on! Food and water fuel every process in the factory – making enzymes, hormones, tissue, energy, nerves – everything. Too little, too much, poor quality or the wrong type of fuel and you reap what you sow - the almost imperceptible degradation of the products produced by your factory – degenerative dis-ease.

There are four steps in the process of fueling the regeneration factory.

1 - Eating and drinking (ingestion),
2 - Breakdown (digestion), delivery of nutrients (assimilation),
3 - Reclamation
4 - Waste removal (elimination).

Important: You can control one of the four steps – eating and drinking – the other three steps are automatic. Once you put food and water in your mouth, the rest of the events are inevitable and occur automatically in your regeneration factory.

The Facts are the Facts. There are two issues to consider at this point of this examination.

First, geneticists are discovering that the number of times that cells can replace themselves is limited. So, if you think you can live forever - think again.

Second, DNA is the recipe for cellular generation and regeneration. Unless there is a DNA anomaly, your factory knows how to produce a cell in the first place and thereafter, reproduce perfect, duplicate cells – each cycle.

Every Cell – Every Seven Years

Deepak Chopra M.D., Ayurvedic Master, author and noted speaker, contends that adults replace every cell in their bodies every seven years during their life.

Your factory literally produces millions of new cells every day to replace those that are failing. If you supply the factory with the appropriate raw materials (ingestion) then each new cell can be as perfect as the original.

On the other hand, substandard cells are produced from sub-standard raw material. Substandard cells make substandard tissue, which makes substandard organs – need I go on?

Simply put, the gradual degradation of the replaced cells creates the almost imperceptible march through the states of well-being - healthy to not sick to sick. At question is the quality of your life during the time you have. While it is a painful subject, I don't know anyone who dreams of suffering through a portion of their life or spending their last years in a nursing home.

Tools Versus Magic Bullets

The supplement industry has changed over the years. Prior to the advent of patent medicine, roots, twigs, leaves, potions and lotions were medicine and self-care – taking responsibility for your own health – was the standard.

Once patent medicine became the norm, people developed a dependence on the science of patent medicine, transferring the responsibility for maintaining and promoting health to others. Unfortunately, the focus for health became reactive – that is taking measures once an individual becomes sick.

People began believing that patent medicine could fix anything and neglected making healthy choices. Supplements were relegated to voodoo. During this dark age of the industry, people sought out these herbal "magic bullets" when there was nothing else that could be done. The fact that there were any benefits at all, given the circumstances, is testament to the body's regenerative ability.

A Renaissance

About 25 years ago, the supplement industry began enjoying a renaissance. Slowly, people started taking responsibility for staying healthy. This renaissance led to an explosion of supplements – bottles of single ingredients – particular vitamins, minerals and herbs.

Unfortunately, all these different bottles of "stuff" frustrated consumers. They knew they wanted to take something, but what? When they left the store, they had a bag full of bottles and a heart full of hope.

Unfortunately, many consumers became frustrated with the daunting task of taking a hand full of pills every day.

Phase Two of the Renaissance

The next phase of the renaissance, nutraceutical supplements, eliminated the frustration of buying and taking hands full of single ingredient supplements. One nutraceutical supplement can take the place of several bottles of pills on your shelf plus, nutraceutical supplements take the risk out of mixing the wrong "stuff" or taking too much of a particular single ingredient. They are convenient, inexpensive and effective because the formulas contain multiple natural ingredients, combined in the right amounts to achieve consumer expectation. The nutraceutical revolution is helping people buy what they want – affordable, effective, natural products.

There's a Problem. It takes time for supplements to work because it takes time for the body to regenerate.

Patience is a virtue - but waiting for a supplement to "kick in" is a significant source of frustration for many people. Consumers do become impatient – and fueled by the aspirin syndrome (i.e., Got a headache, take an aspirin, stop the headache), the consumer becomes disappointed and abandons a particular regimen.

Plus, the lack of short-term results provides the 'Doubting Thomas' proof that - "*Those things can't work! It's just hocus-pocus.*"

The easiest way to stay healthy is to not get sick! But, if you have the misfortune to be experiencing a spiral from health, it isn't the end of the world. Sometimes, a little professional intervention, some fuel for your factory, some time to regenerate and - only time will tell. It all depends on why and how far you've spiraled downward. One thing for sure is that it is never too early, but, unfortunately, it may be too late.

Your Life – Your Choice

I am reminded of a TV commercial for FRAM oil filters that aired in the mid-seventies. It compared the small investment for an oil change and new filter to the cost of a new engine. At the end, the announcer said, "Pay me a little now, or pay a whole lot more later!"

THE REGENERATION FACTORY

The Opportunity of a Lifetime

Imagine a factory that fuels itself, builds all its finished goods from scratch, reuses 80% of its recyclables; heats and cools itself. A factory that automatically repairs machinery; replaces worn out parts and protects itself, day and night. I dare say this technological marvel would be touted as the eighth wonder of the world. Can you imagine the value of the stock of such a company? What if that factory used cheap raw materials to build a product that lasts more than 70 years? Somebody would make a fortune!

Don't expect to read about this marvel in the business section of your local newspaper – it's your body – but it's a marvel just the same. You exist because your body uses inexpensive raw materials: water, protein, fat, carbohydrates, minerals and vitamins to build and operate itself.

The regeneration factory works around the clock, every day of the year, producing millions upon millions of products (cells). This process starts at conception and continues, uninterrupted until death.

Your factory doesn't stop because it can't! The process can't pause either. Even when the factory is supplied with substandard raw material, that rightfully should be rejected in quality control, the process goes on …and on …and on. Descriptions of what constitutes quality raw materials have been detailed, in great lengths, in any number of works. Those are decisions that you must make because once you put something in your mouth, there is no turning back. Suffice it to say that you are what you eat. Those of you who choose to be Ronald McDonald, or to be Colonel Sanders, could do better!

How Your Factory Works

The assembly line starts at your mouth where the raw materials are mixed with enzymes and passed through the esophagus for further processing.

After a brief waiting period, the materials are treated with stomach acids before moving into the intestines to finalize the conversion of the raw material into components that can be used to operate the factory.

The components pass through the intestinal wall and are carried throughout the body by the circulatory system, along with oxygen, to be delivered to specific sites where they are combined, according to a specific set of blueprints that scientists call DNA, to create or rebuild tissue.

Once the new components are delivered and processed at the specific site, the waste is gathered up, returned to the circulatory system where they are carried back to the intestines for elimination. This waste, along with food residues are gleaned for recyclable materials, after which the remainder is expelled from the body.

Your Body's Management Team

Like any efficient factory, there is a management team that is responsible for the entire process. The process is carefully monitored for the availability of components as compared with needs; component deliveries are scheduled and made in a timely manner; workers are trained and deployed.

The brain is the manager, monitoring and directing activity with hormones, which are the messengers. Once a need is uncovered, hormones direct enzymes, which are the workers, to perform a particular task. Hormones measure the performance of the task and, using messengers and workers, report progress to your brain and wait for further instruction. New instructions are delivered back by, you guessed it, messengers and workers...hormones and enzymes. This process, like most processes performed by the body, is ordered. Everything happens automatically except for selecting and chewing food.

Enzymes are the workers in the factory. Virtually everything that happens does so because of an enzymatic action.

Dr. Edward Howell, noted researcher and author of Enzyme Nutrition, The Food Enzyme Concept, identifies three classes of enzymes: 1 - digestive enzymes, 2 - metabolic enzymes and 3 - food enzymes.

He explains that digestive enzymes and metabolic enzymes lose their potency over time and must be replenished by the enzymes that come from the food we eat.

The complication is: food enzymes are destroyed when the food is over cooked or processed. Diets consisting of cooked, packaged and processed foods lack the sources of the raw materials (food enzymes) on which the body depends to maintain the potency of the digestive and metabolic enzymes.

Howell warns that once the reserves of enzyme "raw material" are depleted (due to reliance on a cooked, packaged and processed food diet), digestion and body function is affected. The inevitable, almost imperceptible, degradation of enzyme potency robs people of what Howell describes as *Life Force*.

Everyone should read Dr. Howell's work. Ask your local librarian for a copy. It can change your life: Enzyme Nutrition, The Food Enzyme Concept, Dr. Edward Howell, Avery Publishing, Wayne, New Jersey.

Probiotics are an integral part of the efficiency of the assembly line. Probiotics are friendly organisms that live throughout the intestinal tract. Estimates are that there are more of these friendly organisms existing in the intestines than there are cells in the body.

While the thought that our intestines are teeming with other organisms is perplexing, it is normal and common in our world. Scientists call this relationship symbiosis: the living together of unlike organisms, in close association, when mutually advantageous. These organisms complete the preparation of nutrients for assimilation and, during the process, produce substances and certain vitamins that support immunity.

Probiotics are Essential for Life

Their role cannot be understated because without them, and the work they do, we would cease to exist. Unfortunately, these organisms are vulnerable. Dietary choices, alcohol, agricultural residues and antibiotics affect the populations of these friendly organisms and the mutually advantageous work they perform.

Unquestionably, enzymes and probiotics are essential for the efficient operation of the regeneration factory. Together, they are the one point on which this elegant design depends.

When these processes operate efficiently, radiant health cascades throughout the body. Conversely, the consequences of diminished enzyme reserves and decimated friendly intestinal organisms are experienced throughout the body as well.

One Option

Dr. Howell suggests that one way to maintain enzyme reserves and potency is to eat raw, uncooked, unprocessed food.

In addition, carefully wash all the fresh, ripened fruits and vegetables to remove any and all residues; select meat that is free of parasites and other contaminates which are normally neutralized during cooking.

And, purchasing organic meat and dairy products that are void of agricultural antibiotics, which are introduced during commercial production, avoiding prescription antibiotics and eating generous amounts of soured dairy products such as yogurt, buttermilk, cottage cheese and whey would protect and encourage the colonies of friendly intestinal organisms – probiotics.

Another Way

If the prospects of these choices are unreasonable, there are enzyme and probiotic supplements that are helpful for achieving the same objectives. In either case, the benefits of managing the assembly line of the regeneration factory are essential for radiant health.

Products of the Regeneration Factory

Departments

Every factory has departments that function, in coordinated fashion, to achieve a common goal. The Regeneration Factory does too! Organs, glands and the like are departments operating within the factory to achieve a common goal – growth and regeneration – and, just like departments in a factory, have form and function.

Form & Function

For example: skin could be considered the roof and walls of the factory. Its form is a covering; its function is to contain and protect the factory. The immune system provides security. Its function is detecting and eliminating threats to the factory. The digestive tract is the assembly line. Systems…glands…organs. You get the picture.

Form and function. Sure, there is every sort of specialized tissue and fluid imaginable, but in the final analysis, the issue is form and function.

Exacting Specifications

There is a blueprint and set of instructions, that scientists call DNA, definitively describing the form and function of every cell. When there is a need to grow (make more cells) or regenerate (replace damaged or worn-out cells), the factory workers simply retrieve the blueprint and the instruction manual, go to work and, in short order create a product that is built exactly to specifications.

A Big Job

There is a certain enormity to the task due to the variations of form and function. It may be helpful to think of cells and tissue as brick walls. Just like there are endless variations of brick walls – color, patterns, shapes, styles and height – there are endless variations of cells and tissue: eyes, ears, stomach, joints, etc. And just like a brick wall is one brick held to another with mortar, cells and tissue are one amino acid held to another with minerals (with a few vitamins sprinkled in for good measure).

The variations are endless; researchers have identified 20 different amino acids - the periodic chart contains 109 distinct elements - and there are several vitamins.

Certainly, there is a mathematician that can cipher the number of variations, suffice it to *say the number is big!* It is comforting to know there is a blueprint and instruction manual for each and every brick in the wall.

Something to Behold

The regeneration factory operates around the clock, every day, building an endless variation of products with precise specification, form and function.

Now, that's something!

And it all starts when you decide what to put in the assembly line – your mouth. The factory operates around the clock, every day. It doesn't stop or even pause – because it can't.

Inventory Shortages

What happens when the blueprint calls for something that isn't there? The workers simply turn the pages of the instruction manual to Plan B or even Plan C. Sure, the product isn't as good, but what choice is there?

The burning question is: When it's time to make the same product again, (and there's almost always a next time) are the workers following the instructions for Plan A, B or worse C? Which, by the way, may explain why you don't feel like you used to! Your body is producing too many Plan C's.

Simply Elegant

The elegance of this process can be lost in a mountain of minutia. Amino acids come from protein – which is nothing more than fruit, vegetable and animal tissue – which is some combination of 20 amino acids, 109 elements and a sprinkle of vitamins. *Pretty simple, huh?* That is why nutritionists encourage you to follow the food pyramid – eat meals consisting of servings from each of the various food groups every day – they have components that are contained in the Plan A instructions.

That is all you need to do – in theory. The question is: Are the fruits, vegetables and animals created with Plan A instructions?

Reams of paper have been dedicated to decrying the sad state of our food. The truth is somewhere in the middle – some are created with Plan A instructions, others aren't. Do they have the stuff you need? Some do – Some don't.

Those of you who have the time and inclination to try – congratulations and good luck – your chances are better than those who don't do anything. For the rest of us, there are supplements.

Fueling the Regeneration Factory

Factories operate because they are supplied with energy of some sort: human hands, electricity, coal, oil or natural gas. Your regeneration factory needs energy to operate as well. The difference is your body makes its own fuel from oxygen, water, fat and simple sugars that derived from carbohydrates and plant sources (don't confuse these with refined sugars).

Metabolism is a word that describes the body's fuel consumption. Basal Metabolic Rate (BMR) is the rate of fuel consumption when your body is operating normally.

Metabolism is an ordered, complex reaction: a group of hormones direct a group of enzymes to combine the molecules of oxygen, water, fat and sugar in a particular way, to move the substance into the cell, to explode the substance creating energy, heat and waste and to remove the waste from the cell(a). It may be helpful to think of it as the furnace in your house.

Orderly Process

Just like the furnace thermostat, the body has sensors that monitor the metabolic process so it can be compared to the demands of the factory. The body is able to adjust the speed of the process raising and lowering metabolism. When demand is low, the body disposes of sugar and zaps fat with enzymes that store it for future use. Conversely, when demands are higher, fat is reclaimed from storage to be mixed with sugar for more energy, a process similar to raising and lowering the temperature on the thermostat for a furnace.

When warranted, the body adjusts the octane of its fuel by adding more sugar and reducing the fat in the fuel mix. Instead of burning more fuel, the body simply raises the octane by increasing the sugar content and reducing the fat. (The substance that makes muscles hurt after strenuous exercise, lactic acid, is the byproduct of burning this higher-than-normal octane fuel. Once the "high octane demand" is over, the body processes the byproduct into a substance that can be eliminated, and your muscles stop aching.)

The factory expects a consistent flow of the components for the fuel it needs. Plus, it *puts away a little fat* in case of emergency.

The ability to call on reserves and raise the octane of the fuel is left over from a time when life wasn't as easy – a time when predators necessitated flight, food was seasonal and meals were less frequent. If threatened by a predator, the adrenal system created a spurt of hormones to super-charge metabolism.

When food was not plentiful, the body simply turned down the thermostat to conserve the fat component of the fuel. In fact, your body can choose to protect these reserves even further by using muscle tissue, instead of fat, to sustain metabolism.

OLD ANSWERS – NEW PROBLEMS

Today, we do not need to worry about Saber Toothed Tigers. The new tiger is stress. And just like days of yore, the flight system responds to the threat.

The difference is that today we endure more stress than when our ancestors encountered Saber Toothed Tigers in their day. That, in and of itself, places more pressure on the flight-fight system. The body is being super-charged in response to the perceived threat, stress, more frequently and for longer periods of time. That "spike" places extraordinary demands on the flight response (the adrenal system), affects homeostasis (balance) forcing other supporting systems of the body to compensate. The body needs more fuel – your appetite responds and because of the high-octane requirements, your body wants sugar!

Did you eat an apple today? Noooooo…?

You likely had a Super-Sized Fast-Food Attack! So, your body gets sugar (glucose) for a super-charge (even though it is the wrong kind of nutrition) and your body gets FAT!

Since you're using energy (glucose) like your ancestors did, fat requirements for a source for the fuel mix are constant and, in some cases, lower – ba-da-bing – stored fuel equals stored fat.

Over Fed – Under Nourished

Most of us don't need to worry about our next meal. Instead, we overload the body with fast foods like pizza, hamburgers or the like. Or we skip meals because we have too much to do. Or we just mindlessly nibble away at stuff that can't possibly fuel the body efficiently. Then, we try the latest starvation or carbohydrate or protein diet (pick one). The body senses that high quality food is not plentiful and responds by turning down the thermostat. More fuel, less demand – ba-da-bing – stored fuel equals more fat.

There's a Problem

We are perpetually sending mixed signals to the body's thermostat. Stress, no stress. Starvation, abundance.

The discord wreaks havoc on metabolism.

What to do? Keep the furnace in overdrive risking adrenal overload? Turn down the thermostat risking lethargy? Store fat for the upcoming food shortage? Up … Down. Up … Down. What to do?

Unfortunately, the body generally turns down the thermostat since lower metabolism places less demand on the body. It delivers Store…Store… Store.

There are those who say that Americans are overly concerned with the way they look – that dieting to look good is a preoccupation from which no good can come.

Please, read on. This is important. The number one health problem in America is obesity.

Obesity is defined as about 20 pounds overweight. That's the difference between putting on your blue jeans or struggling to get them on! It is the difference between avoiding the reflection you see in the mirror when you get out of the shower or looking at it.

Think about this: How many people would agree to carry around a sack of potatoes on their back, all day, every day? I dare say most of you would not. If you have carried a baby, a backpack, a large purse, or a briefcase for any length of time, you know it stresses your joints, muscles, and affects your balance and posture.

When you carry around fat you are doing the same thing. Plus, you are asking your body to make and support more skin and tissue; build more arteries, produce more blood and pump it longer distances; inhale more oxygen to support the mass of tissue; build more veins to remove waste; move the wastes further. The entire infrastructure of your body must expand to support carrying around that sack of potatoes – all day, every day.

The National Institute of Health in 1985 concluded that, besides the psychological burdens, obesity increases the risks or severity of many illnesses and decreases longevity.

The American Cancer society found that obese men had higher rates of death from cancers of the colon, rectum and prostate. Obese women had higher rates of death from cancers of the uterus, ovaries, breast (after menopause), gall bladder and bile ducts.

People who are obese (20 pounds or more over normal weight) are more likely to experience high blood pressure, high blood cholesterol and strokes. Adult-onset diabetes is also more common in overweight people (weight reduction may help control inherited diabetes as well).

A New Paradigm

Thermogenics is the science of dealing with the manner in which the body uses dietary calories to produce heat and energy instead of fat.

Obesity research has shown that resetting the body's thermostat adjusts the proclivity to store dietary calories, encouraging it to burn both dietary and stored calories (fat). Other research has pointed to combinations of natural ingredients which may be helpful for supporting thermogenesis.

These supplements, while they are not a panacea, have been helpful with adult weight management when used in conjunction with sensible eating and moderate exercise.

TIPS FOR LOSING WEIGHT

- Set a realistic target.
- Use your head. You know what you should and shouldn't eat. So, eat wisely and moderately.
- "Thirsty" and "hungry" are often confused. Try drinking a glass of water before you start "grazing"!
- Don't give up your favorite foods – eat less.
- Spot special problems like high-calorie snacks, mood-related-eating and special-event lapses (holidays, weddings, etc.)
- Plan ahead – never leave your meals to chance.
- Eat your meals more slowly.
- Avoid second helpings.
- Avoid eating and drinking while watching TV.
- Avoid the cocktail hour and alcohol generally.
- Drink at least 8 - 8 oz. glasses of water each day.
- Get up and start moving. Moderate exercise, like walking, really helps!
- Take your supplements.
- Don't feel guilty – just get back on track.

Look Bad – Feel Bad

Defining "beauty" is a topic for someone else, but the adage, *you feel as good as you look*, merits consideration. Almost everyone who is overweight will benefit from losing their extra pounds, and your heart, lungs and joints would appreciate the help. Plus, wouldn't it be nice to feel good and look great?

Important: Remember, it took time to gain weight, it will take time to lose it!

A NEW BEGINNING

It is interesting to note the changes relating to issues of health between generations.

Earlier generations focused on staying healthy – out of necessity. Today, we have delegated the responsibility for managing our most valuable asset – health – to someone else. Our focus is *– just give me a name for what ails me so someone can give me a pill to fix it.*

Instead of taking proactive measures to stay healthy, we are reacting to illness.

"Eat, drink and be merry 'for tomorrow may never come"!
But what happens when tomorrow arrives?

The problem is that we have stopped making healthy choices. Instead, we wait until we experience the consequences of those choices, hoping for some sort of miracle. And, waiting could be a dangerous business because when you've reached that point, it is a slippery slope. More times than not, there is no magic bullet – no miracle - only the lingering consequences of the choices we have made.

The first thing you must do is understand that there is no one who has more to gain, or lose, than you. The choices you make today have a profound impact on the time you have …and your final years.

- Injuries happen – be careful! Stay fit.
- Infections happen – be careful! Practice good sanitation.
- Degeneration happens – no one is going to live forever.

The second thing you must do is start making healthy choices.

- Start drinking at least 8 – 8-ounce glasses of water every day. Juice, coffee, tea or soda do not count.
- Start thinking about what you put in your mouth.
- Eat a lot more fresh, raw fruits and vegetables.
- Read labels on prepared and processed foods. If you can't pronounce it, either ask someone to explain or look it up.
- Eat breakfast. Toast and coffee is not a good choice!
- Eat lunch. Cut back on fast food restaurants – choose better.
- Eat dinner. Eat early enough to allow for digestion.
- Control your between-meal snacks. If you are eating right, it doesn't matter anyway!
- Start a moderate exercise program. My favorite is a brisk walk!

The Answer Isn't What You Think.

There are those who believe you can get everything you need to stay healthy from the food you eat – if you choose wisely. Perhaps, but not likely.

Dr. Joel Wallach D.V.M., ND, in his book, <u>Rare Earths, Forbidden Cures</u> (Double Happiness Publishing Company, Bonita, CA), explains that commercial agricultural practices deplete the minerals of the soils in and on which the crops are grown.

If the minerals are not in the ground, they are not in the crop.

Harvesting fruits and vegetables before they are ripe, to accommodate transport to market and to extend presentation time in the stores, diminishes their nutritional values.

Storage, cooking, canning and processing reduces the value even further.

"In some cases…", Wallach contends, "…you would be better off eating the package the stuff comes in!"

There are those who believe you can ignore your diet and take supplements. This position evaporates when you inspect the labels…they are called Dietary Supplements – not dietary alternatives.

The likeliest choice should be – ***do everything you can***! After all, your factory works around the clock regenerating itself.

The products it produces can be manufactured from the "A list" components, which provide the factory everything it needs to enjoy the glow of *HEALTH*,

the "B list" components, with *NOT SICK* products that require compensation from systems of the factory,

or the "C list" components which virtually assures the degeneration of the efficiency of the factory – a poor state of health – *SICK*.

Time Heals All Wounds

Regardless of the condition of your regeneration factory, it works around the clock – every day – following the original blueprint – which describes the *GLOW OF HEALTH.*

Providing “A list” components to the assembly line - and time, can regenerate the glow.

It is never too soon to start making better decisions and taking responsibility for your health.

In the final analysis it is you – and only you – who have the most to gain and the most to lose!

The elegant simplicity of your body’s regeneration factory shouldn’t get lost in detail. After all, the easiest way to stay healthy is to not get sick!

IT’S YOUR LIFE – IT’S YOUR CHOICE

Invest in health or spend on declining health and sickness.

ABOUT THIS BOOKLET

Many of my clients said "*People need to know this stuff. You should write a book.*" so, I did. A VIEW OF HEALTH - An introduction to natural health and holistic healing was written to help the reader develop a framework for understanding the elegant simplicity of protecting, maintaining and improving their health naturally.

For some, this short explanation was enough. They took the information and made a difference in their lives.

Others wanted more! So, I wrote, along with one of my clients, Jeanie Traub, CREATING RADIANT HEALTH – Keys to Unlocking the Healing Powers Within.

The book is a hit, too.

It's been called "*The owner's manual you should have received with your birth certificate.*"

Jackie C. A. from Energy Wellness wrote on Amazon "… *I want to thank the authors for such a great & inspiring workbook, it totally changed my life and health. I now own & control my health and overall wellness. God bless!* "

If you want or need more – order the book - Creating Radiant Health. Check out Amazon here for the e-book or soft cover book, or a bookstore near you for your copy.

ABOUT THE AUTHOR

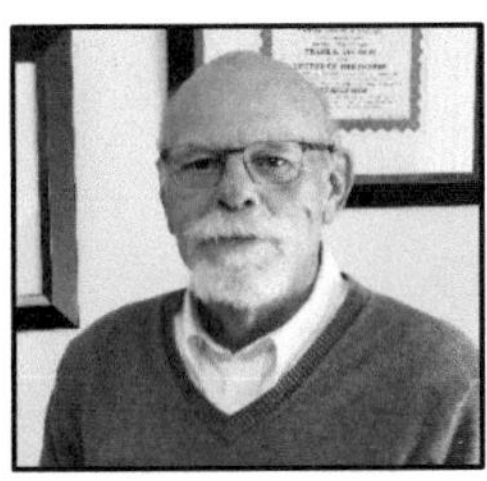

Dr. Frank A. Lucas is not a medical doctor. He has several honorariums, including Certified Natural Heath Consultant (cNHC), Doctor of Philosophy (PhD) with extensive, significant experience in natural health counseling, holistic health and healing, natural medicine, complementary medicine, alternative medicine, and natural remedies.

He has written several holistic, natural health and healing books; published numerous essays and articles; lectured nationally and internationally; and has been featured on several online blogs, addressing current natural health and holistic healing issues.

During three decades of service, Dr. Lucas has counseled thousands of clients with health and wellness issues, helping them identify appropriate alternative therapies and herbal remedies for health problems and conditions and how to incorporate natural medicine, herbal remedies and lifestyle therapies into personal health and wellness plans.

Frank's single-minded mission is to help his clients, and now you, build a lifelong strategy for keeping the body working efficiently, which, in the final analysis, is the bounty of true health.

Printed by Libri Plureos GmbH in Hamburg,
Germany